On Death of a Beloved

- Recovering from loss of a loved one -

On Death of a Beloved

- Recovering from loss of a loved one -

by
Dr. Lloyd Stenbeck

By Dr. Stenbeck

<u>Books:</u>

Healing Yourself -- The Holistic Approach

Heal Yourself Right Now! [The Seven Priority Organ Levels for effective Nutritional Treatment.]

The 22 Unique Body Types!

<u>Booklets:</u>
(Step-by-step details on accomplishing each issue)

  #1 *Start Healing with Positive Thinking*
  #2 *Mastering Positive Feelings for Health*
  #3 *Spiritual Balance and Your Healing*

These books are available on-line at the usual source.

About the Author

Educated in New Zealand and in the USA, Dr. Stenbeck attained B.S., M.S., D.C. degrees (Chiropractic). His holistic healing methods have been profiled in magazines (Esquire, McLean's, Playgirl, the Atlanta Constitution), and on TV in the USA and in Canada. He was the main contributor to the Warner Book, *The Eye/Body Connection*, by Jessica Maxwell, which focused on the holistic healing relationships between the iris structure and organ genetics.

In the 1970-80's, he was elected Fellow, Royal Society of Health, London; Fellow, American Association of Chemists; and Affiliate, Royal Society of Medicine, London. For several years, he produced a TV show in Los Angeles public access called *"The Health Doctors"*. He has practiced in two medical partnerships, where the patients benefited from medical and holistic healing. He is a member of Self-Realization Fellowship. For further information on his on-line consultation, biography and healing methods, see his web site: *DrStenbeck.net*

* * *

The information in this booklet represents a distillation of healing methods acquired from treating patients and from the personal loss of my daughter.

In true holistic healing, we doctors are particularly involved in assessing whether you have any mental, emotional, or spiritual stress overloading into your organs—and these stresses are all capable of causing illness! As you will discern from the following chapters stress sets the stage for tissue irritation or in associated organs.

A classic example is how mental worries and stress irritate the stomach, before proceeding to ulcers or worse.

This booklet provides the steps you need to fake for complete recovery from the loss of your loved one.

You can recover; God and your loved one expect you to recover, so read on and do it!

* * *

Contents

Preface   *viii*

1. *The Premise*   *1*

2. *The Mental Aspect*

    Affirmations for Positive Thinking   *3*
    Health Problems from Mental Stress   *5*
    Nervous System Nutritional Support   *8*

3. *The Emotional Aspect*

    Negative Emotions   *11*
    Acquiring my Positive emotions
    through the Written Release   *14*

4. *The Spiritual Aspect*

    Symptoms of Spiritual Stress   *17*
    Why me Lord?   *18*
    Prayer/Meditation in my recovery   *20*

Appendix   *22*

* * *

On Death of a Beloved

Recovering from loss of a loved one

* * *

1. <u>The Premise</u>

There is no greater loss.

The bond we have with our children is so strong that in an emergency we would instantly give our life to save the child. You know it. Can we ever recover from losing such a beloved? The answer is, yes.

Your soul, spirit, creator, demands and expects that you not only recover from the loss, but that you become happier than ever, just as your beloved would want you to be! You know it is true! The beloved one wants you to recover, get over it, treasure and celebrate the loving memories of their life, and become happy again. Do you think they would want you to stay depressed and miserable for years to come? If you think that, stop reading!

Your healing starts with being aware of your thinking: are you being positive or negative? For your mental *and* physical healing, you must recover your lost positive thinking. I recommend certain affirmations and appropriate nutritional support for this aspect of recovery from your loss.

You then explore the negative feelings taken on from the loss of your beloved, like depression, anger, rage, guilt, loss of intimacy, shame, blame, heartbreak, sorrow, despair, etc.—all of which become sequestered in specific organs thereby contributing to dysfunction of those organs. Also provided is a list of commonly found emotions from loss. A written method of releasing your negative feelings is included, which ensures you manifesting positive feelings and behaviors in recovering from your loss—as your loved one would want for you!

Finally, I address the spiritual aspects of your loss. Some of you will hold lost faith or other feelings about God, which contributes to health problems.

This booklet addresses how to accomplish your recovery, and to be happy again. My patients have done it. I did it after the loss of my daughter. Now you do it.

* * *

2. *The Mental Aspect*

Affirmations for Positive Thinking
Health Problems from Mental Stress
Nervous System Nutritional Support

* * *

Affirmations for Positive Thinking

Mental stress affects you when your intense thinking and worrying—in this instance from the loss of a loved one—exhausts your nerve nutrients; this results in mental stress overloading into your body classically into the stomach, intestine, adrenal glands, lymph, and thymus gland, and threatening the health of these organs.

(See Appendix for Hans Selye's extensive research.)

Your mental body, the part of the nervous system doing your thinking, is quite amenable to being positively or negatively programmed. If you speak *negative* words to yourself about your loss, silently or out-loud, then you are reinforcing the belief of whatever you are saying:

"I am useless."

"It's my fault."

"I have failed."

"I want to die."

"My life is over."

"I wish I was dead."

"I can never recover."

"I should have done... ."

"I'll be unhappy forever ."

Of course, some negative thinking is natural after such a calamity! Just work on minimizing it. Watch your thoughts, and when a negative comes up choose to replace it immediately with something positive.

But—if you speak *positive* words to yourself, then you <u>will</u> believe whatever you are saying and this kick-starts your healing:

"I recover from my loss."

"I am moving through my grief."

"I will always love and treasure (his/her) memory."

"I forgive (him/her) for dying/leaving/ abandoning/betraying me/needing to leave."

"I accept what happened as I slowly but surely recover."

"I find my peace and spiritual center after his/her passing."

"I complete my grieving and become happy again, just as (he/she) would want for me!"

This aspect is the essence of *'affirmations'*, where you speak specific positive words to yourself for reprogramming negative thoughts; this facilitates your 100% mental balance and positive thinking about your loss.

* * *

Doing the Affirmation

Select a positive statement from the above list, or construct your own, that parallels your thinking about the dominant negative thoughts plaguing you from the loss. Then speak the affirmation, out-loud to yourself, repeated twenty-one times, twice daily, for two weeks. After completing it, you will believe the potential truth of it, and the associated health problems will start resolving immediately. (The following section addresses the *Associated Health Problems* of your mental stress.)

You may sometimes need one or two other affirmations after concluding your first choice.

* * *

These health problems start after your mental stress overloads into certain organs (resulting in acupuncture imbalances that precede organ dysfunction):

Stomach, Intestines — irritation or inflammation, ulcers, indigestion, constipation, low back pain, weak thigh muscles; may result in irritable bowel syndrome and related conditions; with relentless stress, death is possible from a bleeding ulcer

Lymph, Thymus (Immune problems) — healing problems, infections, mid-back pain, chest muscle weakness

Adrenal glands — adrenal insufficiency, hypo-glycemia (low blood sugar), moodiness, fatigue, depression, headaches, weak thigh muscles, knee and back pain (see the following Chart)

Less often, other organs and tissues such as the bladder, throat, and esophagus may be involved.

Any healing of the above organs is necessarily incomplete without the appropriate nutritional support of your nervous system. In most instances these organs start healing immediately after attaining mental balance.

* * *

Fatigue
Fainting
Headaches
Cold intolerance
Menses problems
Loss of motivation
Poor healing ability
Sex organ problems
Low blood pressure
Knee pain or weakness
Mood swings or depression
Neck, mid- and low back pain
Dilated pupils, visual problems
Bone, joint, teeth, gums, skin problems
Self: anger, rage, fury, failure, self-failure
More mental stress and negative thinking

The following section addresses the *Nutritional Support* you need for attaining mental balance and positive thinking.

* * *

The following nutritional supplements are essential for restoring mental balance and positive thinking, as you recover from this loss.

Nutrients —

Research shows that severe mental stress depletes certain vitamins and minerals that then impair your nervous system recovery; the result is more mental stress and negative thinking, with consequent health problems. For a general approach to resolving this problem, take these supplements with food:

- *Vitamin B-Complex*: 2 capsules, twice daily, for two weeks; then maintain on 2 capsules once daily for several months
- *Calcium/Magnesium*: 2 capsules, twice daily for a month, and then maintain on 2 capsules once daily; or, *Multi-minerals* (*not* trace minerals) at the same dose as above.

You will probably need this nutritional maintenance for six months to a year, or until recovery is well underway.

<u>*Herbal Support*</u> —

You might regain mental balance without this herbal component, but many people have environmental toxic metal or chemical issues affecting their health (from polluted air, food, and water), and a herb is often needed to adjunctively support your nervous system recovery.

Take one of these herbs, one capsule (or one teabag) twice daily with food, for about three months:

Chamomile, White Willow, or Chickweed

* * *

<u>*Food Support*</u> —

Secondary to the above, consider these dietary aspects:

- Minimize processed and junk foods
- Eat a diet rich in raw fruits and vegetables, salads, whole grains, seeds, and nuts
- Eat moderate protein, 2-4 oz., twice daily of eggs, fish, poultry, meat; (if vegetarian, have 20 gm. daily of a protein drink/shake, in addition to other vegetable protein foods that you eat)
- Stop eating white sugar, corn syrup, and chemical sweeteners

* * *

3. *The Emotional Aspect*

Negative Emotions
Acquiring my Positive feelings through a
Written Release

* * *

<u>Negative Emotions</u>

This section addresses the emotional pain around your loss. Negative feelings must be released, or your health will suffer and recovery from your loss is delayed.

Any number of negative feelings may have hit you. I usually think of these emotions as 'infinite negative feelings' that, because of the intensity of your emotional pain, have turned against yourself as 'infinite <u>self</u>-negative' feelings that then lock into your unconscious mind.

Specific feelings like, loss, grief, betrayal, and abandoned may predominate in your emotional pain (see the following *List* for examples). To make matters worse, the emotional pain downloads into your mental body aggravating your negative thinking around the loss.

To help your recovery from this aspect, I describe a highly effective written release of negative emotions from your mind and body. (Releasing negative emotions is discussed further in my earlier books.) Intense negative feelings may cause a "runaway mind" where negative thoughts run wild creating scenarios of failure and ruin.

Guilt
Despair
Ashamed
Wounded
Desperate
Decimated
Humiliated
Obliterated
Abandoned
I'm a nobody
My life is over
Overwhelmed
There is no God
Fear, dread, terror
I will never recover
I have failed (him/her)
I might as well be dead
There is no hope for me
I've made too many mistakes
God will never forgive my sins
Unreal expectations (it's my fault, etc.)
And the self-component of such feelings.

The following written release of your negative feelings is somewhat related to the release done in the *Twelve Step* programs, with some extra steps. It is a very efficient way to reprogram your emotions, and psychologists I know find it very helpful in their practices.

[Note: If you have cuss words in your mind about your loss, be sure to write them out or the reprogramming will not occur. In most cases, doing each release once is enough.]

Method — Address this writing to God, or to the Universe, or creator, etc.

For the release, in Part A, you write about what happened and what you went through with the loss.

In Part B, insert the feelings you probably went through (have an intelligent guess from the previous List, the reprogramming will still happen). You most likely hold infinite negative feelings (and self-infinite) feelings in your whole being, along with grief or sorrow.

In Part C, forgive your beloved for leaving you (and forgive yourself if you feel guilty for any reason).

In Part D sign and burn the document to release the programming.

* * *

The Written Release

Part A: I write to God about my loss…

Part B: I now release my unconscious negative emotions, negative beliefs, etc.…

Due to: _______________(name)
Locked in my: _______ HEART and whole being
Replace with opposite positive feelings of:
____

Part C: I forgive the person for abandoning me. I now forgive _______ for causing me to suffer, and I ask him/her to forgive me if I ever caused any pain.

Part D: I sign and burn the document

Read the document out-loud. I <u>sign and burn</u> it to facilitate the releasing and removal of the retained negative feelings from my mind and body.

* * *

*Example of a Written Release
of your Emotional Loss*

<u>*Part A:*</u>	*I write about my loss….*
<u>*Part B:*</u>	*I now release…*
Issue:	*overwhelmed, abandoned, heartbreak, and infinite negative (and self-negative) feelings*
Due:	*to my loss of…*
Locked:	*in my HEART and my whole being, and overloading into my mental body causing negative thinking*
Replace:	*100% <u>mourning integrity</u>, and choosing to be <u>happy again</u> (as he/she would want me to be!) 100% <u>accepting</u> what happened as I completely recover (as he/she would want…) 100% HEART and <u>mental balance</u>, positive thinking (as he/she would want of me).*
Part C / D:	*Forgive. Sign and burn document.*

15

I have included some references in the *Appendix* regarding how for several years psychologists have been reporting their research on the efficacy of written releases in emotional and physical healing.

* * *

3. _The Spiritual Aspect_

Symptoms of my Spiritual Stress
Why me Lord?
Prayer/Meditation in my recovery

* * *

Symptoms of my Spiritual Stress

You may experience any of these symptoms from the loss of your beloved causing a spiritual body imbalance:

- Exhaustion
- Weakness in most muscles
- Any unresolved healing problem
- Unable to effectively pray or meditate
- Unable to surrender your pain to God
- Lost faith that you will ever recover from your loss
- Unbelieving in God (higher power, creator)
- Lost faith, trust, or belief in God or a higher power guiding your life

* * *

How could you do this to me God? How could you allow this loss to happen? I cannot forgive you for this? I cannot believe it! Why do I deserve this suffering? And so on...

If you blame God for your loss, do a written release as in the previous chapter, and replace the blame in your whole being with acceptance of what happened as you completely recover.

Such loss of a loved one does cause spiritual stress. We must stop blaming God or the universe for our life problems—otherwise our God relationship suffers. Accept that it happened and *release* all negative programming around God, otherwise we hold negative feelings around the loss, and also around God, causing that relationship to suffer.

An example follows of how to release your negative feelings with God about your loss.

Example of a Written Release around God
(e.g., blame)

<table>
<tr><td><u>Part A:</u></td><td>I write to God about blaming him
for my loss….</td></tr>
<tr><td>
<u>Part B:</u></td><td>
I now release…</td></tr>
<tr><td>
Issue:</td><td>
blaming God for what happened,
and losing faith in him</td></tr>
<tr><td>Due:</td><td>to my loss of…</td></tr>
<tr><td>
Locked:</td><td>
in my HEART and whole being and
overloading into my mental body</td></tr>
<tr><td>
Replace:</td><td>
100% <u>accepting</u> that God did not
cause my loss, and that everyone
creates their own destiny; and
100% restoring my <u>faith</u> in God, and
100% <u>mourning integrity</u>, and
becoming <u>happy again</u> (as God
and my beloved would want for me)
100% <u>mental balance.</u></td></tr>
<tr><td>
Part C/ D:</td><td></td></tr>
<tr><td></td><td>I ask for God's forgiveness.
I forgive my beloved for leaving me.
Sign and burn the document.</td></tr>
</table>

<u>*Prayer/Meditation in my Recovery*</u>

* * *

Consider how prayer will help your recovery. If you believe in life after death, and in God, then pray to God and to the soul of your loved one, by expressing your love. Design a prayer that covers all your needs in recovering from the loss.

Write a love letter to that person who you loved and always will. When finished, sign and burn it, and in some divine way your beloved will receive this letter. You will feel happier knowing your beloved is with God in heaven.

For example:
Dearest......
I love you my dearest one, and I thank you for the love you gave me. I will treasure my memories of you. Your love will always inspire me, and I hope you felt that love from me. Please forgive me for anything I ever did to hurt you, as I forgive you for having to leave me! God needed you back in his arms and I know you will still be there when the time comes for me to join you. I know you must now be in bliss, and that you wish you could have said a goodbye. But we will be together again. We will hold each other again in a spiritually loving embrace. I thank you for having been in my life, and for fulfilling me. Such love I may never know again—until like you, I am with God...

And so on. Express love and gratitude from your heart and soul. Remember your loved one is probably happy to be out of here and back with God!

You might also consider writing a specific love letter that addresses all of the loving memories you have with the loved one, ending it with love and gratitude for the love you received (and sign and burn the letter).

I know of many people, God-loving or not, who after the death of a loved one, report feeling or hearing some sort of communication with the spirit of that person. It has happened to me. It can happen to you.

If you do <u>not</u> believe in life after death, I would suggest you consider doing your own version of the above love letter. It will help you.

* * *

Meditation is always helpful in your recovery as it is about communicating with God. Be quiet, sit and breathe deeply for a while, and then just mentally keep repeating a phrase for 10 or 15 minutes, like:

    "I love you God, I love you, I love you," or

    "Help me to accept that my loved one is safe in your arms," or

    "I thank you for the love he/she brought to me," or…

    "My life has been blessed by knowing him/her," or

"My grief and mourning will pass quickly
knowing he/she is in your arms," or
"I return my grief and mourning to you
Lord, as I am reestablished in your love."

Use your own words to design appropriate loving phrases to meditate on. After the time of your mourning is completed, you will be able to remember the loving good times with your loved one without crying uncontrollably. Some tears may come for the rest of your life, but they will become tears of joy for what you had with your loved one.

Know you will be together again.
God bless.

* * *

<u>*Appendix*</u>

Further Reading:

A. On Mental Stress Healing   24

B. On Emotional Stress Healing   26

C. On Spiritual Stress Healing   29

D. On Contacting the Author   31

<u>A. On Mental Stress Healing</u>

Hawkins D, Pauling L: *Orthomolecular Psychiatry*, Reading, San Francisco, 1973. Classic book on nutritional treatment of mental stress.

Hay L: *Heal Your Life*, Hay House, Carlsbad, CA 1986. An essential aid to forgiveness and self-forgiveness; organ and emotion issues and remedial affirmations.

Holmes TH, Rahe RH: The Social Readjustment Rating Scale, *J Psychosom Res* 11:213-218, 1967. Research on the significant impact of stress on health.

Holmes TH, Rahe R, and others: *The Nose*. An Experimental Study of Reactions within the Nose in Human Subjects during varying Life Experiences, Thomas, Springfield. Shows how thinking of stressful events causes nasal tissue damage.

Pauling L: Orthomolecular Psychiatry, *Sci* 60:265-271, 1968. The Nobel prize winner's work on vitamins and nutrition for healing the mind.

Ponder K: *The Healing Secret of The Ages*, DeVorss and Company, CA, 1966. One of Ponder's many excellent books on mental affirmations in healing.

Selye H: The Story of the Adaptation Syndrome, Montreal: *Acta Inc Med Publ* 1952. Discusses organ reactions to stress. Selye wrote many excellent books on stress, with thousands of scientific articles.

Selye H: *The Stress of Life*, McGraw Hill, NY, 1978.
Essential reading on understanding the
physiology of how stress damages the body.

Simonton O: *Getting Well Again*, JP Tarcher, Inc., 1978. A
classic new age healing work on mind/body
integration.

Tache J, and others: *Cancer, Stress and Death*, Plenum
Press, NY, 1979. Correlation of stress events with
disease.

Viscott D: *The Viscott Method*, Houghton Mifflin
Company, Boston, 1984. Manual for mastering the
stress of life.

Watson G: *Nutrition and Your Higher Self*, Bantam, 1971.
Fascinating account of nutrition and brain function.

Yogananda P: *Where There is Light*, Self-Realization
Fellowship Press, Los Angeles, 1988. Inspirational
Indian saint's work on mastering the stress of life.

B. Emotional Stress Healing

Bradshaw J: *Healing The Shame That Binds You*, Health
Communications Inc., Deerfield Beach, Florida,
1988. This outstanding communicator inspired
millions with his books, PBS specials, and wisdom
about shame and sexual abuse.

Diamond J: *Life Energy*, Dodd, Mead and Company,
NY, 1985. Presents the muscle testing relationships
between emotions, organs and acupuncture pathways.

Diamond J: *Your Body Doesn't Lie*, Warner Books, 1980. A psychiatrist's muscle testing research about emotional stress retention in the thymus.

Foa E, Kozak M: Emotional Proessing of Fear: Exposure to Corrective Information, *Psych Bull* 99:20-35, 1986. Discusses how traumatic memories are disorganized, how treatment requires organization of those memories, and how writing about emotional pain helps this process.

Hay L: *Heal Your Life*, Hay House, Carlsbad, CA 1986. An essential aid to forgiveness and self-forgiveness, organ/emotion issues, and remedial affirmations.

Holmes TH, Rahe RH: The Social Readjustment   Rating Scale, *J Psychosom Res* 11:213-218, 1967. Research on the impact of stress in causing causing tissue inflammation.

Lipsey M, Wilson D: The Efficacy of Psychological, Educational, and Behavioral Treatment. Confirmation from Meta-Analysis, *Amer Psych* 48(12):1181-1209, 1993. Demonstrates the health benefits from writing about emotional pain.

Matarazzo JD, and others: *Behavioral Health*, John Wiley, NY, 1984. Early work on emotions, personality, and health.

Pennebakker JW: Putting Stress Into Words: Health, lingustic, and Therapeutic Implications, *BehaveTher* 31: 539-548, 1993. Evolving research on the efficacy of written releases for negative emotions.

Pennebakker J, Smyth J: Telling One's Story:
Translating Emotional Experiences Into Words
as a Coping Tool. In: Snyder CR (Ed.), *Coping: The
Psychology of What Works*, Oxford University Press,
NY, 1999. Provides a theoretical framework for
understanding how writing about traumatic
experiences resolves negative memories.

Selye H: *The Stress of Life*, McGraw Hill, NY, 1978.
Essential reading on understanding the
physiology of how stress damages the body.

Smyth J: Written Emotional Expression: Effect Sizes,
Outcome Types, and Moderating Variables, *J Consult
Clin Psych* 66:174-184, 1998. How emotional writing
about traumatic incidents produces great health
benefits.

Smyth J: Written Disclosure: Evidence, Potential
Mechanism, and Potential Treatment, *Adv Mind-
Body Med* 5:161-195, 1999. Presents evidence that
written emotional disclosures produce health benefits.

Stone A, and others: Writing About Stressful Events
Produces Symptom Reduction in Asthmatics and
Rheumatoid Arthritics: A Randomized Trial, *JAMA*
81:1304-1309, 1999. Compelling evidence of health
improvements through writing about emotional pain.

Sudakov KV: *Emotional Stress and Arterial Hypertension*,
American Publishing Company, New Delhi, 1983.
Evidence for emotions as a primary cause of disease.

Van der Hart, O and Op den Velde, W: Traumatic
memories. In: van der Hart (Ed.), *Trauma, Dissociation,
and Hypnosis*, Lisse, Swets & Zeitlinger, The
Netherlands, 1993. Evidence for writing about
emotional pain and deconditioning traumatic memories.

Van der Kolk, B and van der Hart, O: The Intrusive Past:
the Flexibility of Memory and the Engraving of
Trauma, *Amer Imago* 48:425-454, 1991. This work
shows how emotional trauma affects memories.

Viscott D: *Emotional Resilience*, Crown Trade
Paperbacks, NY, 1996. His final book: an excellent
work on emotions and illness.

C. Spiritual Stress Healing

Bach E: *The Bach Flower Remedies*, Keats Publishing, Inc.,
New Canaan, 1979. Bach's research on spiritual
imbalances and repressed emotions in healing.

Buscaglia L: *Love*, Ballantine, NY, 1982. One of several
inspiring books by this charismatic teacher.

Cayce E, *Furst J* (Ed.): Story of Attitudes and
Emotions, Berkley Books, NY, 1976. Metaphysical
components of emotions, attitudes and illness.

Gerber R: *Vibrational Medicine*, Bear and Co., Santa
Fe, New Mexico, 1996. An absolute classic
presentation of energy medicine, energy fields, and
healing.

Joy MB: *Joy's Way*, St. Martin's Press, NY, 1978.
Physician's spiritual methods of healing disease.

Locke S: *The Healer Within*, Dutton Books, NY, 1986. Good
introduction to self-healing.

Ponder C: *The Dynamic Laws of Healing*, DeVorss and Co,
LA, 1966. Ponder, a devotee of philosopher Emmet
Fox, on affirmations that change your life.

Scott Peck M: *The Road Less Traveled*, Simon and Schuster, NY, 1978. The highly inspirational book on integrating psychology and the spiritual life into your healing.

Yogananda P: *Where There is Light*, Self-Realization Fellowship Press, LA, 1988. Most writings by all the Indian saints are inspiring and helpful.

* * *

D. Contacting the Author

For further information, or to comment on this book see my web site: _DrStenbeck.net_

You can always email me from the website if you require more help with your healing.

* * *

www.ingramcontent.com/pod-product-compliance
Lightning Source LLC
Chambersburg PA
CBHW070059260726
48658CB00002B/907